ADHD Partners

The Path to Embracing Life and Awakening Personal Power

KIMBER NELSON, CPC, ACC

Copyright @ 2017 by Kimber Nelson

All rights reserved.

No part of this book may be reproduced, in whole or in part, in any form or by any means electronic or mechanical, including photocopying, recording, or by any information storage and retrieval system now known or hereafter invented, without written permission from the author. Permission requests should be sent to the contact page at:

www.ADHDPartners.com

For ordering information, requests for Kimber to speak to your group, or to learn more about setting up private coaching session, contact Kimber through the contact page at:

www.ADHDPartners.com

ISBN-13: 978-1977782014

Introduction

"To raise new questions, new possibilities, to regard old problems from a new angle, requires creative imagination and marks real advance in science."

Albert Einstein

Smart guy, that Albert Einstein.

Why would a ADHD and relationship book start out with a quote from a scientist? Don't worry, you are in the right place.

If you have done any research at all on ADHD (and I am betting you have) you understand that when ADHD shows up many of our unconscious default expectations and perceptions go out the window.

Our friend Albert forgot to mention one key piece, solid information is required for us to have a strong base to launch our new questions, possibilities and perspectives and mark our advance in life and relationships.

Fair Warning:

This book is not your typical book about your partner's ADHD. It is not even about ADHD....not really (although it is packed with information on how ADHD shows up in relationships).

This book is for you, the partner without ADHD.

Navigating the roads of ADHD that you were not aware existed at the beginning of your relationship.

Riding the waves of emotion that are complex and tangled

Hitting the realization that the relationship that you thought you had during courtship looks very different in the day to day business of living

Searching for understanding of things in your relationship that you have not been able to be make sense of…which led you to this book.

ADHD had been described as having a "race car brain"

It's no wonder that Non-ADHD Partners often feel like "they have one foot on the gas and one foot on the brake."

How do you manage this sometimes gear-grinding feeling? Stay focused on taking action. Stay Beautiful. Stay Tenacious.

Welcome to ADHD Partners. You are in the right place.

The Time Is Now

Support for the non-ADHD Partner can no longer be overlooked. You might be having feelings of isolation, anxiety, eroded self-esteem, and mistrust of your own perceptions and your decision-making capabilities.

Understanding how ADHD shows up in your relationship is the first step towards taking back control of your life and relationship.

The second step is utilizing your new-found perspective to empower yourself to act on the things you can control (there are more than you think).

In this book, you will be introduced to my Quadrant Coaching model which breaks down the overwhelming challenges you are facing into powerful bite sized pieces that move you forward. You will rediscover yourself and grow newly discovered strengths as you work through each Quadrant.

The 4 Quadrants are:

- ✓ Connecting – The Connecting Quadrant focuses on acknowledging that with knowledge comes power, supporting you in moving from feelings of being blind-sided and confused to focused on the things that you can control in life and your relationship.

- ✓ Releasing – The Releasing Quadrant creates understanding of how expectations are colored by the societal perceptions of ADHD tendencies and internalized relationship rules, and allows releasing these of these assumptions.

- ✓ Balancing – The Balancing Quadrant brings to light common feelings experienced by non-ADHD Partners such as isolation, overwhelm, and challenges with trusting themselves and others. Over time self-esteem is eroded and forward movement is stalled.

- ✓ Creating – The Creating Quadrant looks at new relationship boundaries and partnership agreements, and places self-care and support back as non-negotiable priorities.

QUADRANT 1:

THE CONNECTING QUADRANT

THE CONNECTING QUADRANT

ADHD impacts every aspect of life. To truly understand the unique and often unexpected paths it takes in your relationship, you need to first understand how it shows up day to day for your partner.

Impulse Control

This can manifest as impulse spending that creates financial difficulty, getting sidetracked and being late to events, impulsively going on a tangent and forgetting a commitment that your partner made to you.

What is one area in your relationship that is impacted by your partner's challenge with impulse control? There may be several broad areas, but I would like you to identify one specific interaction that you can expand on later.

Poor Follow Through

Poor follow through can be connected to many ADHD traits. Regardless of why it happens, it can create a ton of tension in your relationship.

This can also cause an imbalance in the relationship, shifting it from an equal partnership to parent/child dynamic.

Future Awareness

People with ADHD have trouble connecting the present moment to the future. Being able to fully live in the moment is likely one of the things that you appreciate about your partner, but it can create issues as well.

A big project coming up may be put off until the last minute (because it isn't NOW yet), which leads to deadlines missed and work submitted far below what they are truly capable of.

Time Sense

Our definition of time sense is the ability to subconsciously be aware of the passage of time. This can include not noticing the passage of time while being sucked into the rabbit hole that is the internet.

It also encompasses difficulty estimating the time it takes to drive to work (or completely neglecting to include travel time into the morning schedule at all), which creates chronic lateness.

Short Term Memory

Short term memory issues impact following through on commitments. Your partner may simply be forgetting that they agreed to do something that you asked.

Short term memory can also cause challenges with solving math equations and other processes that require multiple steps.

Emotional Regulation

Many people with ADHD have trouble regulating emotion. This may show up in your relationship as your partner's emotional responses seem "larger than life" and out of proportion to what is occurring.

Some people say that they feel flooded with emotion, and it truly does feel like everything else is overwhelmed by the intensity of the feeling.

Emotional Overload

Emotional overload is a common experience that someone with ADHD has trouble managing on their own.

The difficulty regulating emotions, challenges with prioritization, a tendency to view things "big picture" and trouble breaking that down into details small enough to act on are just a few factors that can lead to this.

Emotional Self Protection

Years of being told that you are not living up to your potential and that you just need to try harder takes a toll on the self-image.

Many people with ADHD spend an extraordinary amount of effort trying to project a social face of having it all together while under the surface feeling that they are anything but together.

Close personal relationships threaten that cover. It is a constant battle between a fear of rejection if these challenges are exposed and having a close, trusting relationship.

Self Protection in Communication

Self-protection tendencies will often show up as a barrier to communication.

Avoiding painful topics by redirecting or simply not engaging is common. Additionally, deflecting with anger or projecting undesirable traits onto their partner may also be a self-protection strategy.

Impulse Control in Communication

Impulsivity can also damage communication. Impulsive tangents will often derail important conversations so it feels like there is never resolution.

Interruptions also make the non-ADHD partner feel unheard and unimportant.

Hyperfocus

Attention issues do not just show up as being easily distracted.

They also create the lesser known hyperfocus, which tends to show up when a person is very interested in a project.

Time sense goes completely out the window along with awareness of other priorities, and it is very difficult to transition out of. Some people show frustration and irritability when pulled out of a hyperfocused state.

Hyperfocus Role in Relationships

It is very common for hyperfocus to be part of an intense courtship and then the attention to move somewhere else.

This can leave the non-ADHD partner questioning the love and commitment in the relationship and experiencing feelings of being abandoned.

You may fall into a cycle of taking negative actions to catch and keep your partner's attention for a short time. This also feeds the impression that they don't care about your feelings until they are at an intense level.

What You Look for You Find

As I mentioned earlier, this quadrant is about becoming more aware of ways ADHD shows up in relationships.

The more aware you are of all the different places that ADHD has been "hiding" in your day to day interactions, the larger the perspective shifts will be. Our goal is to illuminate those dark, hidden corners that up until now have likely confused and frustrated you.

We have focused on understanding the challenges that ADHD brings. I am now challenging you to closely examine the negative perceptions that you have had of your partner up until now. You will discover several areas of conflict ADHD impacts that both you and your partner were previously unaware of.

Look for a positive trait that your partner possesses and share your appreciation for it with them.

This positive may even be ADHD related!

Connecting the Dots

We have covered several ways that ADHD impacts on people and their relationships, and I am sure you have had many lightbulb moments. Take the time to answer the reflection questions below:

What situation comes to mind that an ADHD behavior came into play what you were not aware of at that time?

What key AHA moments did you have?

What perception shift will be most valuable to you going forward?

How will you use these perception shifts to create a better outcome?

What other scenarios are you now aware of that were impacted by ADHD which you did not understand at the time?

Prefer worksheets? Download the worksheets related to these exercises at: www.ADHDPartners.com

QUADRANT 2:

The Releasing Quadrant

The Releasing Quadrant

In this section, we look at expectations and how they are colored by the societal perceptions of ADHD tendencies and internalized relationship rules, and allows releasing these assumptions.

Releasing The Brules

"Brules" are bullsh*t rules that we have unconsciously absorbed throughout our lives.

Vishen Lakhiani of Mind Valley coined the term "brules" for the cultural norms of our society that we often forget to question whether they are limiting us or serving us.

Brules are created to simplify the world so we don't have to live consciously. They are often passed down generation after generation and accepted as how life "should" be lived. Often, we don't stop to consider why things are done a certain way.

The world has vastly changed from the way our ancestors lived, so the way we live should too. Sadly, if you are paying attention to the unconscious rules that you are playing by then you are likely working with rules that are not serving you.

They are actually blocking you from living your best life and showing up as your best self.

I can think of no place that unconscious brules beat us down more than within a relationship with ADHD in the mix. ADHD brings with it a different view of the world and a different way of working in it.

Take a moment and think about all the unconscious "shoulds" that up until this point have shaped what you expect out of your relationship. These "shoulds" come from family, religion and society in general. Then inject what you know about ADHD into the mix, and you will discover a whole new set of brules.

To get you started, here are a few examples:

- ✓ The man "should" make more money than the woman.
- ✓ You "should" end up with a white picket fence and 2.5 kids.
- ✓ The woman "should" do housework and the man "should" do yard work.
- ✓ You "should" work a 9-5 job.
- ✓ You "should" always clean the house before you do something enjoyable.
- ✓ You "should" spend X number of hours a week volunteering or at church.

I am not suggesting that you throw away every rule you currently live. I want you to be aware of those rules and make conscious decisions on which of those rules support the best version of yourself and your relationship.

Measuring Stick

As children and young adults, we often imagine what our relationship will look like when we grow up. These images are gathered from a child's view of adults that they look up to as well as books, TV and movies.

Prince Charming and happily ever after. White picket fences. How we will magically have it together as adults? True love means being able to read each other's mind. There are no conflicts so big that they can't be easily wrapped up in a half an hour show.

At the end of the day... true love conquering all.

Don't get me wrong, I am certainly a fan of the notion that love conquers all. What they don't talk about in the fairy tales is the work and compromises required for happily ever after.

The mind reading ability that magically occurs when you really love someone in fictional movies? It is just that – fiction. So are the childhood images and expectations that we place on our partner and the requirement that we should have a happy relationship.

Just as we dragged our brules out into the light, we are now dragging out the expectations we have within the relationship that are causing conflict.

The Measuring Stick exercise helps us evaluate how important realistic priorities and expectations are to the health of our relationship.

Think about an expectation that you have of your partner that often leads to conflict:

✓ What is the expectation?

✓ Why is it an expectation?

✓ How do you decide if the expectation is met?

For most of us, our reaction when an expectation is not met it is far from pretty. What does your typical reaction look like?

Now place that expectation on the Measuring Stick on a scale of 1-10, your current level of expectation being at a 10.

The expectation of taking out the trash will look something like this:

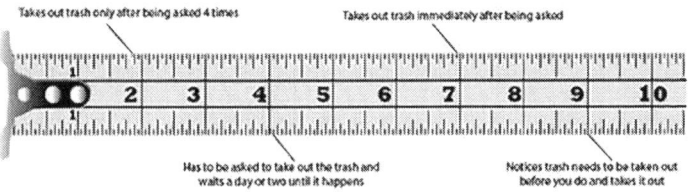

Define what each number on the scale would look like. Take the time to think through each number and be as specific as possible.

To meet the expectation on our example, your partner would need to notice that the trash was full and take it out before you asked to fully meet expectation and get a 10.

Now we go back over each level and evaluate the cost of conflict versus the cost of completion. Note the number that corresponds to the feeling of having this expectation satisfied that is worth the cost of conflict if it is not met.

In our example, it is worth creating conflict in the relationship when our partner does not notice that the trash is full and no action is taken until asked multiple times. When the trash is taken out after being asked once with only a slight delay we count that as a win and not worth damaging the overall health of our relationship.

Most people are surprised to discover that their number is in the 5-6 range. In the past they have pushed for and accepted conflict when a 10 was not met.

What Do You Need?

In the last section, we discussed how to measure where our break-even point is. Break-even is the point where we can be happy with an expectation being met; anything higher on the Measuring Stick is a bonus.

I asked you to measure several expectations so you will have a lot to work with. If you have not done that yet, go back and measure at least 2-3 expectations before you read further.

If you reflect back on how people with ADHD work differently, it will be crystal clear how expecting your needs to be magically known and met is a recipe for disaster!

Now we are going to start getting clear on what your core needs actually are so that you can articulate them to your partner.

Choose the Measuring Stick from the last section that most often causes conflict with your partner. On the number that you circled as your break-even point, underline the items that are critical to that point on the stick that made you decide that it was no longer worth conflict over.

Write those items on a new paper, take a deep breath and go deeper. Ask yourself:

- ✓ What do I feel when this specific item is not fulfilled? (Hint: it is often more about not being heard, respected or valued than how clean the kitchen is.)

- ✓ Knowing what you know now about ADHD, how likely is it that your partner taking (or not taking) that action is tied to the feelings they have for you?

- ✓ If it is related to an ADHD challenge, how can you release the emotional charge that you have previously held when you related that action to how your partner felt about you?

- ✓ Are there already things that your partner does in their own unique way that shows that they hear, respect or value you?

- ✓ What specific actions would help build those feeling? How might you communicate them differently so you get a different result?

- ✓ Remember – in Quadrant Coaching we only focus on what we can control.

What we do control is:

- ✓ Speaking up and asking for what we need
- ✓ How specific our requests are
- ✓ What tone we use when we make a request
- ✓ What language that we use when we ask
- ✓ When we choose to make the request

After you have done everything that you have control over, take a deep breath and let go of any expectation of how your partner responds. If one of your needs is to have a more equal relationship, you must allow the space for your partner to step into.

Note: Specifics are helpful so you are both clear on what that need looks like, but be careful to not fall into micromanaging and sweating the small stuff. Micromanaging, or trying to control your partner's reactions, is a common trap.

Your partner will never know what you need and what makes you feel loved if you don't communicate with them. With ADHD and things like short term memory challenges in the mix, alternate ways of communicating may also be needed – don't give up!

Try different things until you start seeing traction.

What Is Your Small Stuff?

Up to this point we have evaluated a lot of expectations and measured our true break-evens versus the expectation of perfection in most things. Chances are you have had a few light bulb moments and are taking action to create shifts on the things that you can control that are building into big impacts.

Today we are going to do some house cleaning and get rid of the brules that we have been carrying around that are not serving us and the expectations that are really not worth the energy that they are taking up.

My question to you is: What is your small stuff?

It is easy to slip into living unconsciously, functioning like a robot as you move from one expectation to the next and not stopping to question why?

By now, you should have more clarity around some of your whys. But don't be surprised that you uncover more as you increase your awareness of how you live.

Ready?

Good! Now that you have your whys, you can move out of your unconscious robot living with the Rocking Chair Test.

The Rocking Chair Test is a simple yet very effective way to check in on how congruent your life is. When our whys don't match the values we hold closest to us, the mismatch creates frustration, stress, and other unpleasant feelings. When we are living unconsciously, we can never quite pinpoint the source of these jarring, incongruent emotions. However, they start to dissipate once we begin to take actions that are more in alignment with our values.

ROCKING CHAIR TEST

Imagine that you are in last year of your life. You are sitting in a rocking chair on a wide porch with the warm sun shining on you and a slight breeze blowing. You close your eyes. Think back over your life and relationship. Notice what feelings come up.

Happiness? Regret? If only? Why did I?

If the negative emotions around certain tasks or expectations seem out of proportion from the end of life view, then you have just identified your small stuff!

Actively work on letting go of those small things that are causing conflict but at the end of the day are not that important. Focus on what brings more joy, connection, support and love into your life.

What you focus on grows.

QUADRANT 3:
The Balancing Quadrant

The Balancing Quadrant

Now we are shifting to explore common feelings experienced by non-ADHD Partners such as isolation, overwhelm, challenges with trusting themselves and others. Over time self-esteem is eroded and forward movement is stalled.

Trusting Others

Trusting others is essential to the human experience and to connecting at a level that is food for the soul. Society in general is not always conducive to building trust which causes challenges in building any relationship that is deeper than surface level.

Romantic relationships that involve ADHD prior to diagnosis and education often have enormous trust issues. This is due to the perception of ADHD traits through the lens that society have set out, such as:

- ✓ "If he cared about me, they would have paid attention and remembered."
- ✓ "If this relationship is as important to her as she says, then she would have made sure that was done."
- ✓ "He knows this is would cause me issues so I thought I could trust him to follow through in at least this."

Trust can also be severely damaged by the self-protective habits we talked about earlier that may people with ADHD have developed. These habits include projecting faults onto their partner, minimizing and negating the partners hurt feelings, and redirecting the conversation to focus on aspects where blame can be pointed elsewhere. Many people automatically and unconsciously jump so deep into self-protection mode that they are unaware of how these habits negatively impact their partner.

Self Esteem

In Quadrant 1, we talked about several reasons that people with ADHD experience low self-esteem. That is important to understand as it impacts the actions and lack of action that happens in a relationship.

However, it is equally important to understand that when ADHD is part of a relationship, the dynamics involved often create self-esteem challenges for, you, the non-ADHD partner.

Yes, I know… you are "fine"; you will "get by".

But guess what? You are reading this because getting by is no longer good enough.

Living in the land of "Fine" is exhausting, and you deserve better. It is time to get real. We can only create real change when we are real about what is happening now.

Prior to understanding ADHD, it felt that your partner did not hear you. It felt as if they did not care enough to keep commitments. It felt as if they were more interested in getting to know and spending time with strangers than you.

Now that you have a better grasp on how ADHD shows up, you may still feel that way and that is okay.

Because now you know. You know that it is not about you. You know that it has more to do with ADHD than your partner's feelings for you. You know those actions have no direct correlation to how important and valuable you are to them.

So, next time those feelings creep in, challenge yourself to open up and take your new perspective into consideration.

See what happens. It's going to be good.

Emotional Overload

Non-ADHD partners are often the "helpers" of the world who tend to over extend themselves for others.

They can also be very empathetic, which leads to taking on the emotions of those who they are supporting as their own.

Connecting with an ADHD partner who has trouble with emotional regulation and experiences feelings with such intensity that they take over the world can be especially problematic for empathetic helper partners.

The tendency of a helper is to minimize their own feelings about a situation and focus on supporting the other person through their emotions. Therefore, a close relationship with someone who frequently expresses intense emotions takes just as large of a toll on the non-ADHD partners as it does on the person with ADHD (if not more because people with ADHD can often forget or disconnect from the past – sometimes the "past" is just yesterday).

Diminishing your own feelings in an effort to support your partner, while done with the best of intentions, creates an unequal relationship and feelings of being personally diminished, not to mention, the often talked about parent/child dynamic that many ADHD relationships fall victim to due to the ADHD partners challenges with prioritization and follow through.

Many non-ADHD partner end up taking on many of the un-fun "adult" responsibilities which creates an additional unbalancing of the relationship.

Where does your inner helper show up in your relationship?

Trusting Self

In addition to the previously mentioned trust issues with others in the course of a relationship with a partner who has ADHD, non-ADHD partners often start having difficulty trusting themselves and their intuition.

It is common to be told by the most important person in their lives that they are to blame for issues in the relationship. Their feeling are not acknowledged by their partner due to their partner's self-protection tendencies.

When helper tendencies show up, the non-ADHD partner buries emotions themselves due to the intensity of their partner's feelings in the moment.

When you add to these dynamics, don't forget that up until now your perception of what is happening was challenged every day.

It is confusing to look into your partner's face and see that they are earnest in their intentions and then the actual follow through does not match. This is compounded by your partner's reaction when asked about the commitment they made. Self-protection or simple unawareness (prior to ADHD education) often leads to responses that also did not feel congruent with questions were asked of them.

How can you start listening to and trusting yourself, starting TODAY?

Isolation

One of the most common and damaging reactions to the dynamics in an ADHD relationship is for the non-ADHD partner to isolate themselves from family and friends.

This may not be a physical isolation, but an emotional and mental one. You may feel that you are unable to talk to others about what you are experiencing because they won't understand.

At the stage of pre-diagnosis and becoming educated on ADHD, it is extremely difficult to talk to friends and family about the challenges you are facing.

You are confused and having trouble explaining the challenges to yourself in any seemingly rational way so it is understandably difficult to explain to others.

Your friends and family also are lacking the perspective to accurately assess the information. Their typical reaction is often along the lines of telling you that your partner is just a jerk and not worth your time.

This often leads to feelings of wanting to protect and defend your partner and shying away from future conversations because intuitively you know that there is more to it than that. (Although, we all have our jerk moments from time to time. We are certainly not excusing those!)

Add to the mix that many people with ADHD are very good with surface social interactions and present a very put together "social" image. Family and friends will have difficulty reconciling the person that they know on the surface with the difficulties that you share that are underneath the surface.

After a few interactions like these, it is a normal reaction to not put yourself through that again. These experiences can also contribute to self-doubt and not trusting your instincts and your perceptions of the interactions with your partner specifically and the world in general.

What is one way you can re-connect to your community or discover your new community?

QUADRANT 4:
The Creating Quadrant

The Creating Quadrant

Finally, we are ready to look at new relationship boundaries, new partnership agreements and placing self-care and support back as non-negotiable priorities.

It Takes a Village

Have you heard the saying "It takes a village to raise a child?" I am going to expand that to:

"It takes a village to create a successful ADHD relationship."

Now, that does not mean that I am suggesting that everyone in your village/community be involved in every detail of your relationship. However, the fairy tale of a partner in any relationship being the only one able to fulfill all your needs is not accurate.

It is unrealistic to look to another person to fill any internal "holes" that you may have (only you can really do that).

When you are unrealistic about what your partner with ADHD is truly capable of, you are setting yourself up for disappointment.

This is not to negate the value of your partner; this is to set yourself and your relationship up for success. If you are not feeling heard in your relationship due to your partner's attentional issues, work on improving communication and other ways to bring you closer.

At the same time, if you know that there are certain subjects that your partner is going to always have challenges with focusing on, find other people in your community who share that same passion, and include your partner in some of the social aspects of that passion that are more realistic for them to be involved in.

Make the conscious choice to detach from any negative emotions attached to thoughts of what you previously thought a partner "should" do.

Most critically, find your village of other non-ADHD partners who understand what you are going through. It is very empowering to not have to try to justify or over explain what you are going through and the emotions that you are having.

Eyes Wide Open

Living without an understanding of how ADHD impacts your relationship is like finding your way to the kitchen in a large strange house in the dark.

Those critical components that are missing had you stumbling around: disoriented, confused and likely bruised by the end.

You can't control that the large end table with sharp shin endangering corners has been placed in your path. You can control whether or not you continue to battle your way through the dark to the kitchen or focus on finding the light switch that will change your view.

An understanding of ADHD and the shifts in perspective it brings shines the spotlight on those dark corners (and dangerous end tables!) but it is just the beginning.

Take what you have learned and keep focusing what you can control, and the world will continue to brighten!

Self Care

Remember when we talked about the tendency for non-ADHD partners to be helpers by default?

It is hard to argue that being a helper is a bad thing. However, I will argue that one of the pitfalls of being a helper is the tendency to neglect self-care.

Consistently putting your needs second to others will drain you dry until there is nothing left to give.

Before we go further, I want you to take a minute and write down all of the justifications that just come into your mind on why you CAN'T make self-care a priority.

Not enough money. Not enough time. You are dealing "okay" and people you care about need it more. Those are habitual justifications that are keeping you running on empty and without the energy and motivation to show up as your best self—for yourself AND for the ones you love!

While money and time constraints may be real, self-care does not have to take enormous resources:

- ✓ Finding your village is self-care
- ✓ Asking for your needs is self-care

- ✓ Clearing out 10 minutes to walk to the park and enjoy nature is self-care
- ✓ Taking a bubble bath is self-care
- ✓ Adding more fruits and veggies to your diet is self-care
- ✓ A daily 5 minute YouTube meditation video is self-care
- ✓ Discovering a new hobby and making it a priority to learn is self-care

You are worth it!

Creating You 8.0

Initially, I had the title of this section as Creating You 2.0 but that did not quite feel right. Life is a journey, rediscovering yourself or finding who you really are for the first time is a path that takes a lifetime.

Technology goes through numerous reinventions of itself, each version better than the last but often with some unexpected bugs.

Companies know that no matter how much testing they put the product through, there will still be bugs discovered once it is released to the public. Once they become aware of the bugs, they start working on the release of the next version.

Keep moving forward, acknowledging and being aware of bugs while finding the best path around them, often discovering new and better versions of an aspect of life along the way.

Don't forget to give yourself credit for what you are achieving and a break from expectations of perfection.

Expecting a perfect 10 in all things creates unnecessary stress, and let's be honest, it would also get pretty boring!

This work allows you to show up as your best self, the real you that has been buried under the clutter trying to get out. Creating the best you is simply finding the real you that has been there all along.

The Real You 8.0

Thank you for allowing me to be part of your journey!

I hope you received a lot of valuable insight from this small but mighty book. ADHD Partners is a labor of love for me. Love for myself, my loved ones and now you.

*** Please Leave a Review ***

I can't overstate how important these reviews are to making sure other people get a chance to discover ADHD Partners and launch their own Journey into self-discovery. I would also love to hear your thoughts.

Want More?

Head on over to www.ADHDPartners.com and download the worksheets that accompany the exercise in this book (plus a few bonus worksheets just for fun!)

If you are ready to step into action and work with me, contact me directly at Kimber@ADHDPartners.com to check on availability and details on how to be accepted into the program.

Find us on:

Facebook www.facebook.com/ADHDPartners

LinkedIn www.linkedin.com/in/kimbernelson/

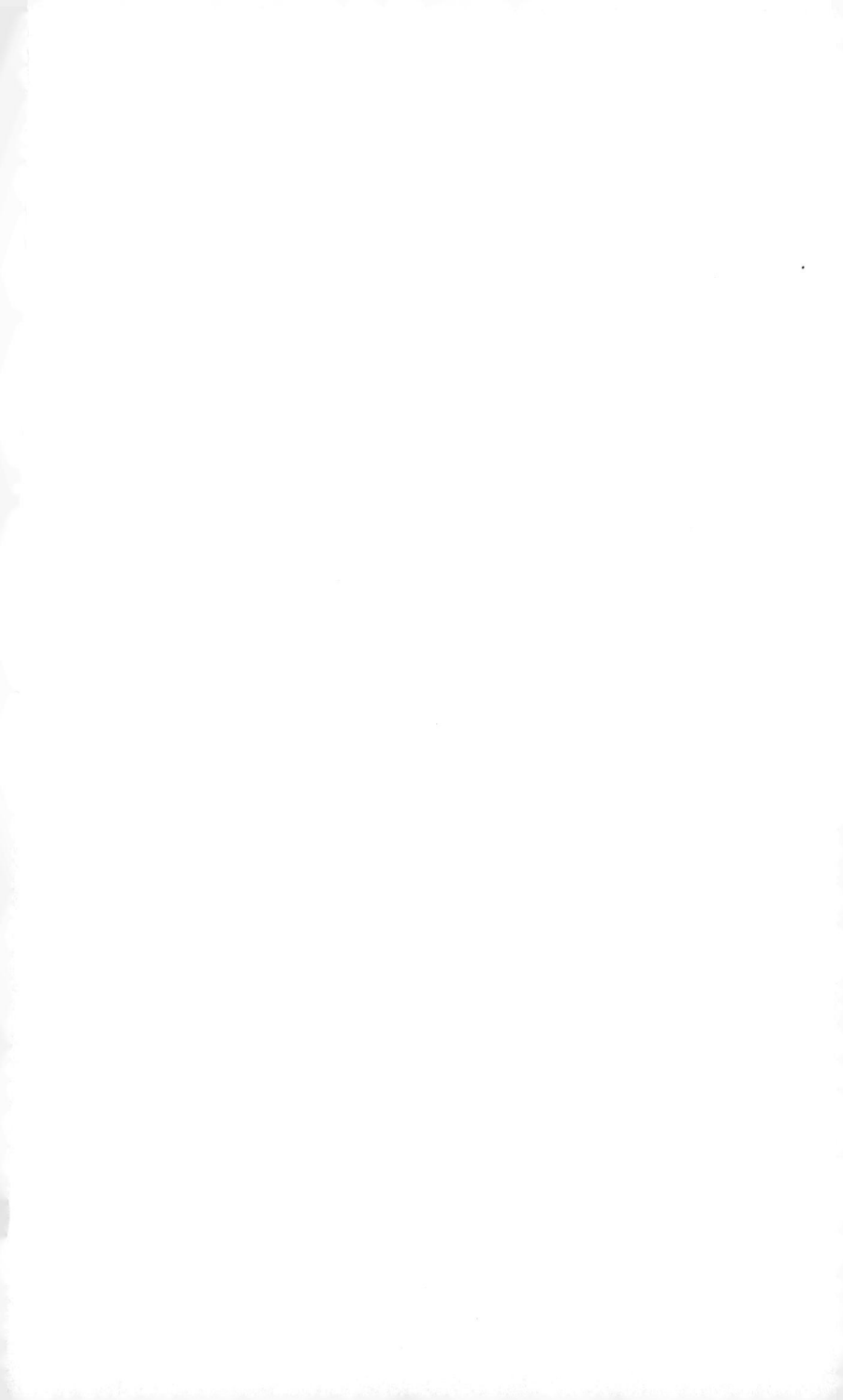

Printed in Great Britain
by Amazon